BEYOND THE PLATE
The Impact Of Mindful Eating On Your Overall Well-being

GLEN ROBERT

Table of contents

Chapter 1

Understanding Mindful Eating

It is important to first have an understanding of what mindful eating comprises before we proceed to discuss its advantages. To put it another way, it entails paying undivided attention to the here and now as well as the act of eating without passing judgment on what one is doing. It's about slowing down and appreciating each meal, engaging all our senses in the experience. By doing so, we become completely aware of our body's hunger and fullness signals, enabling us to eat in a manner that fulfills our physical requirements.

Mindful eating is not merely a fleeting fad or a fast remedy for weight reduction. It is a technique that has profound origins in ancient knowledge and current science. It builds upon the ideas of mindfulness, which entails being present and non-judgmental in the moment. In the context of eating, it involves bringing awareness to our thoughts, emotions, and bodily sensations when we eat. It's about listening in to our body's cues and eating with purpose and attention.

What is Mindful Eating?
Mindful eating goes beyond the sheer act of ingesting food. It is a means of nurturing our bodies and spirits. It is about building a healthy connection with food and ourselves. When we practice mindful eating, we become aware of the deep links between our emotions, thoughts, and food patterns.

Imagine sitting down to a meal and relishing each mouthful. You take the time to enjoy the colors, textures, and tastes of the meal in front of you. You notice the feelings in your mouth when you chew and swallow. You pay attention to the emotions of fullness and contentment that come while you consume. Mindful eating is about being present in these times, without distractions or judgments.

The Origins of Mindful Eating

Mindful eating has its origins in ancient Buddhist teachings that promote attention and attentiveness in all areas of life. The discipline of mindfulness has been handed down through centuries, helping people to live with purpose and awareness. It was popularized in the West by Zen teacher Thich Nhat Hanh and nutritionist Jan Chozen Bays, who realized the significant influence that mindful eating can have on our total well-being.

Thich Nhat Hanh, a prominent Buddhist monk, regularly preaches the significance of mindfulness in all parts of our lives, including eating. He teaches that by being completely present and aware as we eat, we may shift our connection with food and build a greater feeling of appreciation and joy.

Jan Chozen Bays, a physician and mindfulness instructor, realized the need for a mindful approach to eating in our contemporary culture. She witnessed how thoughtless eating had become the norm, leading to overeating, emotional eating, and other bad behaviors. Through her practice, she has led many people to reconnect with their bodies and build a more balanced and nutritious relationship with food.

Together, Thich Nhat Hanh and Jan Chozen Bays have called attention to the crucial feature of mindful eating. They have shown us that it is not only about what we eat but how we consume. By practicing mindfulness at the dinner table, we may convert our meals into times of self-care, nutrition, and self-discovery.

Chapter 2

Mindful Eating: A Path to Mental Well-Being

In the rush and bustle of contemporary life, when time seems to slip away in the blink of an eye, the notion of mindful eating emerges as a guiding light toward overall well-being. It transcends the basic act of eating food, urging us to relish the richness of each moment and create a deep connection between body and mind. In this inquiry, we untangle the transforming link between mindful eating and mental health, revealing the possibility of a more fed and peaceful lifestyle.

Defining Mindful Eating

At its root, mindful eating is a discipline that transcends the mechanical action of placing food in our mouths. It urges us to be completely present, engaging our senses and consciousness in the process of eating. Mindful eating is a shift from the autopilot mode that frequently defines our connection with food, prompting us to appreciate tastes, textures, and the sense of sustenance.

The Mind-Body Connection, and Awareness of Emotional Eating

As we go into the core of mindful eating, we find the delicate dance between the mind and body. This exercise fosters a heightened awareness of physical sensations, building a deeper connection with the messages our body gives. By tuning in to how our body reacts to various meals, we establish the groundwork for a more intuitive and attentive approach to eating. One of the major consequences of mindful eating is in its capacity to bring awareness to emotional triggers for eating. By practicing awareness during meals, people may discern between bodily hunger and emotional needs, stopping the pattern of utilizing food as a coping tool. This heightened emotional awareness becomes a cornerstone for building a better connection with both food and one's own emotions.

Stress Reduction, and Breaking Free from Unhealthy Patterns
In a society where stress is a constant companion, mindful eating emerges as a strong remedy. Slowing down the pace, enjoying each mouthful, and being completely present at meals may have a tremendous influence on stress reduction. The act of mindful eating causes a relaxation response, encouraging a feeling of peace that goes beyond the dining table into our everyday lives. As such, mindful eating becomes a beacon of hope for people suffering from disordered eating practices. By bringing mindfulness to the process of consuming food, people may break

conflicting cognitive patterns connected with eating, promoting an optimum and balanced connection with nutrition. This approach supports a break from rigorous norms and enables an investigation of intuitive eating.

Fostering Positive Relationships with Food, and Practical Implementation in Daily Life
Beyond the physical act of eating, mindful eating helps to the formation of an ideal and sustainable relationship with food. It enables folks to enjoy the nourishing characteristics of food, developing appreciation and respect for the nutrition that powers our bodies. This adjustment in viewpoint may have a cascading impact on self-esteem, body image, and general mental well-being. In this vein, making mindful eating a part of our everyday practice doesn't need a major change. Simple habits such as paying attention to the colors and textures of food, chewing carefully, and enjoying each mouthful may pave the way

for a more attentive approach. Creating a suitable setting, free from distractions, significantly improves the experience of mindful eating.

Beyond the Plate
The influence of mindful eating goes well beyond the plate. It becomes a way of life—a mindfulness practice that informs our everyday decisions relating to diet and self-care. By adopting mindfulness in all facets of our lives, we build a holistic feeling of well-being that transcends the act of eating and penetrates our whole existence. Mindful eating is not simply a technique; it's an encouragement to live with purpose and awareness. As we relish the tastes of our meals, we also savor the moments of our existence. In this trip, we realize that mindful eating is not just about what we eat but how we eat, building a profound connection between body and mind. By accepting this transforming practice, we start on a journey toward a more balanced,

nourished, and harmonious existence—one mindful mouthful at a time.

Chapter 3

Food for your mood: How what you eat affects your mental health

It's commonly recognized that diet plays a crucial part in your physical health. But studies also demonstrate that diet directly influences our mental and emotional well-being, too.

"It makes sense that what we put in our body would also impact our mental health," says Dr. Deborah Fernandez-Turner, Deputy Chief Psychiatric Officer at Aetna. "Good health describes a condition of optimal well-being. That implies the body and the intellect, acting in harmony. Both are equally crucial when establishing your health journey."

The science underlying food and mood
The connection between nutrition and emotions arises from the intimate contact between your brain and your gastrointestinal system, frequently termed the "second brain."

Here's how it works: Your GI tract is home to billions of bacteria that impact the synthesis of chemical molecules that continually transmit signals from the stomach to the brain. Two common examples of this are dopamine and serotonin.

Eating nutritionally rich food encourages the development of "good" bacteria, which in turn favorably influences the synthesis of these compounds. When production is ideal, your brain gets these good signals loud and clear, and your mental state may reflect it.

On the other side, when manufacturing goes astray, so may your mood.

Sugar, in particular, is regarded as a key driver of inflammation. It nourishes "bad" bacteria in the GI tract. Ironically, it may also trigger a transient rise in "feel good" hormones like dopamine. "You don't want that either", adds Dr. Fernandez-Turner. "These spikes result in a fleeting sugar rush, followed by a hard crash."

When you adhere to a diet of nutrient-rich foods, you're setting yourself up for fewer mood swings and an enhanced ability to concentrate. Studies have even discovered that clean diets consisting of largely complete, unprocessed foods, might aid with symptoms of sadness and anxiety. Whereas poor diets have been related to an increased risk of dementia or stroke.

Foods that help you be healthy

So, what should you put in your basket and on your plate? Here's a brief rundown of things to look for next time you're at the grocery shop.

Whole foods

Some research demonstrates that preservatives, food colorings, and other chemicals may induce or aggravate hyperactivity and depression. "If you have one thing to remember, it's to eat genuine food, or food that's little processed and contains a few nutritious ingredients," says Sarah Jacobs, holistic nutritional consultant and co-founder of The Wellness Project. Think fresh fruits and veggies in a range of hues.

The potent nutrients supplied by colorful produce offer loads of advantages for the mind and body. Their nutritional qualities are frequently included in the colors themselves. By including naturally colored foods in our diet, we make it much simpler for our bodies to receive more vitamins and minerals and enjoy the numerous physical and psychological advantages.

Fiber Plant-based meals are abundant in fiber which helps your body absorb glucose (food sugars) more slowly. This helps you prevent sugar surges and crashes. Fiber-rich foods include fruits, vegetables, and nutrient-filled carbohydrates like whole grains and legumes.

Antioxidants

These inflammatory fighters are notably numerous in berries, leafy green vegetables, spice turmeric, and meals rich in Omega-3 fatty acids, like salmon and black chia seeds. Dark chocolate also includes antioxidants — and sugar – so enjoy it in moderation.

Folate

This sort of B vitamin assists with dopamine synthesis without causing it to rise the way carbohydrates do. Find it in leafy greens, lentils, and cantaloupes.

Vitamin D

Vitamin D assists in the creation of serotonin, and we normally receive it via exposure to sunlight. But mushrooms are another wonderful source, Jacobs explains. If you're lacking in vitamin D, your doctor may also prescribe taking a supplement. Aetna members may earn savings on supplements; check your plan's benefits for information.

Magnesium

This vital mineral assists with everything from neuron and muscle function to having a regular pulse. But it's also crucial to the food-mood link. A mineral deficit may harm the flora in your stomach and create sadness and anxiety-like symptoms. Load up on natural sources such as cacao nibs, almonds and cashews, spinach, and other dark leafy greens, bananas, and beans.

Fermented foods

Fermented foods are rich in probiotics, which are particular living bacteria that are excellent for your digestive system. Examples include sauerkraut, kimchi, miso, tempeh, and the fermented drink kombucha. These foods also tend to be heavy in sodium, so take them in moderation or avoid them completely if you have high blood pressure.

Incorporating good-for-your-mood items into your diet may require some additional work at first, Dr. Jacobs notes. She advises preparing a week's worth of chopped vegetables and soaked and cooked beans ahead of time. This makes DIY dinners easy to whip up and just as enticing as take-out. Strapped for time? Dr. Fernandez-Turner proposes utilizing frozen fruit and vegetables and 10-minute brown rice, quinoa, or whole-grain couscous.

You may also try making tiny healthy dietary adjustments, such as swapping white rice, pasta, and bread for whole-grain equivalents. This helps boost healthy fiber in your body, which benefits digestion. And instead of a bag of chips, pick a side salad filled with nuts, seeds, and colorful veggies for added taste.

Of course, standard dietary recommendations still apply. This involves keeping hydrated, not skipping meals, and being aware of your coffee and alcohol consumption. Dr. Fernandez-Turner says. "It's a good idea to discuss with your doctor if you should drink caffeine or alcohol based on your personal health history and goals, and if so, how frequently to stay healthy," she says.

You don't have to feel compelled to make all of these adjustments right now, Dr. Fernandez-Turner points out. "You may find it easier to take things a day at a time or implement a new substitution each week," she adds. For example, one week you might substitute manufactured sugar with fresh fruit, and the following week you could add extra veggies and lean protein. "There's no one-size-fits-all when it comes to your health," she says.

Being present and conscious as we eat is another helpful skill that helps battle cravings or overeating. "Try to notice the way your food smells, tastes, and feels as you eat it," Dr. Fernandez-Turner adds. And take notice of how the healthful snacks and meals make you feel afterward. Some individuals who convert to a largely plant-based diet, for instance, typically realize that their energy and attention are maintained throughout the day.

It may take days or weeks before you start to experience the mood-boosting advantages of a healthy diet. It depends on how many modifications you make. Lasting change doesn't happen overnight, but the healthy choices you make each day build on each other. In time, you'll notice the good consequences in both your mind and body.

Chapter 4

Your brain on food

Think about it. Your brain is constantly "on." It takes care of your thoughts and actions, your respiration and pulse, your senses - it works hard 24/7, even while you're sleeping. This implies your brain demands a steady source of fuel. That "fuel" comes from the meals you consume - and what's in that fuel makes all the difference. Put simply, what you eat directly influences the structure and function of your brain and, eventually, your mood.

Like an expensive automobile, your brain performs best when it receives only premium gasoline. Eating high-quality meals that include plenty of vitamins, minerals, and antioxidants nourishes the brain and protects it from oxidative stress — the "waste" (free radicals) created when the body utilizes oxygen, which may harm cells.

Unfortunately, much like an expensive automobile, your brain may be destroyed if you take anything other than premium gasoline. If chemicals from "low-premium" fuel (such as what you receive from processed or refined meals) reach the brain, it has limited capacity to get rid of them. Diets heavy in refined sugars, for example, are damaging to the brain.

In addition to impairing your body's management of insulin, they also cause inflammation and oxidative damage. Multiple studies have established an association between a diet heavy in refined sugars and poor brain function – and even a worsening of symptoms of mood disorders, such as sadness.

It makes sense. If your brain is deprived of good-quality nutrients, or if free radicals or destructive inflammatory cells are circulating inside the brain's contained area, further adding to brain tissue damage, effects are to be anticipated. What's remarkable is that for many years, the medical community did not fully understand the relationship between mood and eating.

Today, thankfully, the expanding area of nutritional psychiatry is discovering there are numerous repercussions and links between not just what you eat, how you feel, and how you eventually behave, but also the sorts of bacteria that dwell in your gut.

How the things you consume affect your mental health

Serotonin is a neurotransmitter that helps regulate sleep and hunger, control emotions, and decrease pain.

Since around 95% of your serotonin is created in your gastrointestinal tract, and your gastrointestinal tract is lined with a hundred million nerve cells, or neurons, it makes sense that the inner workings of your digestive system don't simply help you digest food, but also guide your emotions. What's more, the activity of these neurons — and the creation of neurotransmitters like serotonin — is heavily regulated by the billions of "good" bacteria that make up your gut microbiome.

These bacteria play a crucial part in your health. They protect the lining of your intestines and guarantee they create a strong barrier against toxins and "bad" bacteria; they reduce inflammation; they increase how effectively you absorb nutrients from your meals; and they activate neurological connections that run directly between the gut and the brain.

Studies have compared "traditional" diets, such as the Mediterranean diet and the traditional Japanese diet, to a typical "Western" diet and have found that the risk of depression is 25% to 35% lower in people who consume a traditional diet. Scientists explain this discrepancy because these traditional diets tend to be rich in vegetables, fruits, unprocessed grains, and fish and shellfish, and include only minor quantities of lean meats and dairy. They are also absent of processed and refined foods and sweets, which are hallmarks of the "Western" eating pattern. In addition, many of these unprocessed foods are fermented, and so work as natural probiotics.

This may seem improbable to you, but the theory that healthy bacteria not only impact what your stomach digests and absorbs but also affect the degree of inflammation throughout your body, as well as your mood and energy level, is gaining momentum among academics.

Chapter 5

How Mindful Eating Affects the Brain

Neuroscientific research has demonstrated that mindful eating engages the prefrontal cortex, the region of the brain responsible for decision-making and impulse control. This activation encourages healthier food choices and helps break away from autopilot eating patterns.

When we practice mindful eating, we engage our brains in a purposeful and aware way, enabling us to make choices that match with our long-term health objectives. By paying attention to the tastes, textures, and sensations of each mouthful, we may relish our meals and avoid mindlessly swallowing unnecessary calories.

Additionally, mindfulness activities have been reported to lower stress and anxiety, further encouraging a better connection with food. By bringing mindfulness into our eating patterns, we may develop a more tranquil and balanced approach to sustaining ourselves.

It is crucial to emphasize that the advantages of mindful eating extend beyond the physical world. By being more attentive to our bodies and the messages they tell us, we may develop a greater sense of self-awareness and self-compassion. Through this practice, we may create a stronger appreciation for the food we consume and the nutrients it gives.

How to Practice Mindful Eating

Now that we understand the advantages and science behind mindful eating, let's investigate how to implement it into our everyday life.

Creating a Mindful Eating Environment

Start by providing a peaceful and pleasant setting for your meals. Set the table, avoid distractions like devices, and create a tranquil setting. Engage your senses by presenting your meals in an artistically pleasant way and using appealing plates and utensils.

Mindful Eating Techniques

Begin each meal by taking a calm, deep breath and appreciating the nutrients in front of you. Engage your senses while you eat - notice the colors, textures, and fragrances of your meal. Chew gently and relish each mouthful, savoring the tastes and textures. Pause sometimes to check in with your body and analyze its state of hunger and fullness.

Incorporating Mindful Eating into Your Daily Routine

Start small and progressively build up your mindful eating habits. Begin by picking one meal or snack each day to eat thoughtfully. As you feel more comfortable, consider adding mindful eating to additional meals. Remember, the aim is growth, not perfection. Be gentle with yourself and exercise self-compassion along the process.

Chapter 6

Benefits of eating Mindfully

Mindful eating is more than a fad; it's a transforming method that connects you with your eating experiences, promoting a healthy connection with food.

It's about being present at meals and paying attention to the tastes, textures, and feelings of what you consume. This practice delivers significant advantages for both your mental and physical well-being.

Embracing mindful eating is embracing a healthier, more connected lifestyle. It's a practical, accessible tool anybody can use to optimize their relationship with food and increase general well-being.

Let's investigate how this simple exercise may bring tremendous improvements to your mind and body.

What are the advantages of eating mindfully?

Certainly, let's look into the incredible advantages that mindful eating brings to the mind. This technique goes beyond the plate, impacting your mental well-being in fundamental ways:

Stress reduction

Reducing stress with mindful eating is attainable and transformational. Instead of blindly hurrying through meals, try these practical strategies to add serenity to your eating experience:

Start your meal with a deep breath. It indicates to your body that it's time to rest and enjoy.

Pay attention to the fragrance, colors, and textures of your meal. Engaging your senses anchors you in the current moment.

Savor each mouthful, chewing carefully. This methodical pace delivers a message to your body that you're sustaining it, minimizing stress reactions.

During the day, take small thoughtful pauses, concentrating on your breath and letting go of stress.

Be cognizant of emotions when eating, addressing them without food as your main outlet.

Enhanced emotional well-being

Enhancing emotional well-being via mindful eating is a profound adjustment that anybody can embrace. Here's how it may favorably affect your emotions:

Mindful eating teaches you to identify the relationship between your emotions and your food choices. It allows you to choose meals that promote your emotional well-being.

By paying attention to your body's hunger signals, you're less likely to resort to food as a coping method for stress or emotional upheaval. This leads to healthy emotional reactions.

Mindful eating cultivates self-awareness, helping you recognize and handle unpleasant emotions more efficiently. It gives a toolkit of better-coping options beyond food.

The practice of mindful eating increases self-compassion. You learn to treat yourself with care, even when confronted with emotional obstacles.

When you appreciate your meal and eat with mindfulness, you lessen the chaotic surge of emotions that might emerge from rapid, thoughtless eating.

Improved concentration

Improved attention is one of the many advantages that mindful eating can bring. When you participate in this exercise, you're not simply replenishing your body; you're improving your attention and mental clarity:

By eating slowly and thoughtfully, you build a pattern that helps your brain to absorb information more efficiently. This may boost your capacity to remain interested in projects and sustain attention.

Mindful eating helps you let go of distractions. When you eat with focus, you're less likely to be cognitively scattered, leading to increased mental clarity.

The practice builds a better connection between your mind and body. This heightened awareness might help you tune in to your thoughts and focus more efficiently.

As stress levels fall with mindful eating, your mind feels more at peace, making it simpler to focus on activities without the interruption of stress-related distractions.

Better decision-making

Embracing mindful eating may lead to improved decision-making in numerous facets of your life. Here's how this exercise may enable you to make more informed choices:

Mindful eating helps you to make deliberate choices about what you eat. This focus continues beyond the dinner table, helping you make informed decisions in all aspects of life.

By being in sync with your body's hunger and fullness signals, you'll develop stronger self-control when it comes to eating. This increased discipline might flow over into other areas, such as handling urges and temptations.

The awareness gained via eating may enhance your problem-solving abilities. You'll become competent at analyzing circumstances and making choices with clarity.

Mindful eating urges you to prioritize your health and well-being. This change in emphasis may lead to a more balanced approach to decision-making, with better regard for your long-term objectives.

Enhanced body-mind connection

Enhancing the body-mind connection is a fundamental advantage of mindful eating. It's about bridging the gap between your physical and mental well-being, leading to a more harmonious and comprehensive life experience:

Mindful eating encourages heightened awareness of your body's cues, such as hunger and fullness. This awareness extends to other physiological feelings, letting you identify when you're tight or exhausted.

With a stronger body-mind connection, you're more prepared to notice and control emotions. You'll gain the skill to react to emotional triggers with mindfulness and self-compassion.

Mindful eating fosters intuitive eating, where you accept your body's clues to guide your food choices. This trust extends to your total well-being, enabling a more intuitive approach to life choices.

As you check in to your body while eating, you become more attentive to bodily feelings and well-being. This heightened body awareness may lead to better living choices.

A healthy body-mind link fosters a balanced view of health and well-being. It helps you comprehend that well-being involves physical and mental components, impacting your whole attitude to self-care.

What are the advantages of eating healthily for the body?

Let's investigate the tremendous advantages that mindful eating brings to your health. This practice goes beyond merely relieving hunger; it feeds your body in ways that might lead to greater physical health:

1. Weight control

Achieving and maintaining a healthy weight is a frequent desire for many. Mindful eating is a realistic method that may enhance your weight control efforts:

Mindful eating helps you become attentive to your body's hunger cues. You'll learn to eat when hungry, eliminating overeating prompted by environmental stimuli.
When you eat deliberately, you relish each mouthful, finding pleasure in fewer servings. This may naturally lower calorie consumption.
Mindful eating emphasizes resolving emotions without resorting to food for

solace. This interrupts the loop of emotional eating and encourages healthy coping mechanisms.

The technique corresponds with intuitive eating, where you trust your body's instincts to guide food decisions, eventually promoting a healthy weight.

2. Improved digestion

Enhanced digestion is a fundamental advantage of mindful eating. Here's how this technique may help to greater gut health:

Mindful eating fosters a slower pace, providing your body more time to break down food properly. This may alleviate stomach pain and bloating.

When you eat consciously, you tend to chew food more completely. Proper chewing is a vital stage in digestion since it initiates the breakdown of food in your mouth.

Mindful eating may help decrease stress levels, which is crucial since stress can adversely affect digestion. Reduced stress improves digestion.

Savoring your food and savoring each mouthful may lead to a more relaxed eating experience. Stress-free eating aids improved digestion.

Mindful eating enhances the link between your mind and body. You become more aware of how various foods influence digestion, leading to more educated dietary decisions.

Mindful eating supports balanced dietary choices, including fruits, vegetables, and whole grains. This balanced diet is helpful for intestinal health.

3. Nutrient absorption

Efficient nutrient absorption is a vital part of general health, and mindful eating may considerably contribute to this process:

Mindful eating promotes you to make mindful, nutrient-rich dietary choices. This ensures your body obtains the critical vitamins and minerals it needs for optimum operation.

By paying attention to your meals and concentrating on a range of foods, you ensure a balanced diet. Different foods supply different nutrients, boosting total nutrition absorption.

When you eat slowly and carefully, your digestive system performs more efficiently, absorbing nutrients effectively from the food you ingest.

Mindful eating entails understanding your body's water demands. Proper hydration is crucial for vitamin absorption since it helps carry nutrients through the body.

4. Balanced blood pressure

Maintaining balanced blood pressure is vital for general health, and mindful eating may assist greatly in accomplishing this goal:

By lowering stress associated with rushed or thoughtless eating, this technique may aid in reducing blood pressure levels.

Mindful eating enhances awareness of portion sizes, limiting overeating, which may lead to hypertension.

Paying attention to the salt level of meals may lead to lower sodium consumption, an important element in blood pressure management.

Mindful eating creates a nutrient-rich diet, promoting overall cardiovascular health and blood pressure control.

5. Better sleep patterns

Achieving healthier sleep patterns is a desirable effect of practicing mindful eating:

Mindful eating avoids heavy or stimulating meals close to bedtime, favoring a calm condition suited to sleep.

Eating carefully may lessen the chance of nocturnal indigestion or discomfort, allowing for unbroken sleep.

By minimizing stress associated with hasty or emotional eating, mindful eating may increase sleep quality and duration.

Recognizing your body's water demands, an element of mindful eating helps reduce nightly awakenings due to thirst.

Consistent meal timings and mindful eating may help synchronize your body's internal clock, supporting regular sleep-wake cycles.

Mindful eating is not only a nutritional strategy but a habit that may dramatically enhance both your mind and body. It's about establishing a more thoughtful and conscientious relationship with food, and by implication, with yourself.

So, I urge you to engage on this journey of mindful eating, not as a rigorous regimen, but as a road to a more thoughtful and meaningful existence. By enjoying each mouthful, listening to your body, and making mindful decisions, you're not only feeding your body but also building a deeper connection with yourself.

Chapter 7

Overcoming Challenges in Mindful Eating

While the advantages of mindful eating are great, it's crucial to understand and solve the problems that occur along the road.

Common Obstacles and How to Overcome Them

One typical difficulty is the inclination to eat on autopilot or in reaction to external stimuli like commercials or emotions. Developing awareness of these triggers is the first step in resolving them. Cultivate mindfulness in your everyday life beyond meal times, since this will help you become more receptive to your body's signals and feelings. Additionally, seek encouragement from loved ones or join mindful eating groups to keep motivated and exchange experiences.

Maintaining Motivation for Mindful Eating
Staying motivated in any activity demands dedication and reminders of the advantages. Reflect on the good improvements you've experienced in your physical and emotional well-being. Practice self-compassion and remember that mindful eating is a process, not a destination.